SUPER HEALTH IN STRESS ENVIRONMENT

DEDICATION

Asher and Benjamin. Grow in grace and multiply in strength. Dip your feet in oil. Dwell in safety and in wisdom without limits.

ACKNOWLEDGMENT

The team at the Plantrician project. Thank you for the gift of a "life-time" conference in the summer of 2017. For the privilege to meet for the first time, Dr. Dean Ornish, and being in the same room with the likes of Dr. William Lee, Dr. T. Collin Campbell, Dr. Caldwell Esselstyn and several other Plant-based Nutrition Practitioners from around the world. It was indeed a turn-around moment for me, and an opener to what possibilities exist in reversing and managing conditions through plant-based nutrition.

Thanks to the team that worked on this project.

Foreword

Studying the requirements for healthy living will always bring to mind the words of the Canadian Clergyman, A.J. Materi, *"So many people spend their health gaining wealth, and then have to spend their wealth to regain their health"*.

It is fast becoming a truth that the price of success can be very demanding as we journey on in life, especially for those born without the proverbial "silver spoon". Sometimes, the price paid takes a toll on our health, a price some people pay with their own lives.

This work is to help individuals working the hours and going the extra hours yet want to stay healthy. It will deliver into your hands easy and quick suggestions on how to combine a busy schedule and maintain a health balance.

The dietary advices are practicable and will help anyone go through the day feeding on the important nutrient factors as required by the body, for health and proper aging.

Above all, Dr. John Christopher said in his book, "Curing the Incurables", that there are no incurable diseases but there are only incurable people. This book might be the solution to the issues tagged incurable in your health.

INTRODUCTION

Longevity potential has decreased with time for humans despite the increase in knowledge and landmark breakthroughs in technology and modern medicine.

Economic realities have reduced the attention given to diet and nutrition while interventions have become substitutes instead of alternatives.

Commercial advertisement has not really helped in the choice of what to feed on and how to live, with many people largely ignorant and unwilling to take responsibility for their health.

The need to make ends meet has become the decisive factor in determining what to eat, where to live and how to live for a larger portion of the population globally.

Working conditions, especially in developing economies with weak labor laws have become a critical link to ill-health in recent times.

The purpose of this book is to identify quick-wins to help individuals who spend about 4 hours on the road to work 10 hours daily.

Stress is the underlying factor of many diseases and can be prevented if properly managed.

"So many people spend their health gaining wealth, and then have to spend their wealth to regain their health."

- A.J. Materi

CHAPTER ONE
STRESS AND STRESS ENVIRONMENTS

When the body undergoes pressure and conditions not normal to its intended design, our nervous system and adrenal glands, because of the body's intelligent design, send signals to the rest of the body, in readiness for a physical response.

This is a basic instinct that we have evolved to help us cope with potentially dangerous situations, and is known as the "fight or flight" response.

Stress is the body's system of response under inappropriate pressure. This response may sometimes alter normal body activities, stimulating responses with symptoms like palpitations, dizziness, indigestion or heartburn, tension, headaches, aching muscles, trembling or eye twitches, diarrhea, frequent urination, insomnia, tiredness, impotence, etc.

Stress also has a considerable impact in the workplace. The workplace is one of the several stress environments. The UK's government agency, The Health and Safety

Executive, says there is a convincing link between stress and ill health.

Its research with *Personnel Today Magazine* recently showed that over 105 million days are lost to stress each year, costing UK employers £1.24 billion. The research is based on responses from almost 700 senior HR practitioners and almost 2,000 employees.

Other findings include:
- 11% of absence is attributed to stress
- 52% say stress is increasing
- 60% claim stress is damaging staff retention
- 83% think stress is harming productivity

Workplace stress can cause organizations to lose millions of pounds through high levels of absenteeism, long term absence and a dwindling productivity amongst staff.

Pressure itself is not bad as individuals sometimes thrive on it. Problem starts when those pressures exceed a person's ability to cope.

The human body responds to stress mentally or physically, which in turn affects the person's emotion and physical well-being.

As stated above, not all stress is bad. Good stress is called **eustress** while bad stress is referred to as **distress**. Stress becomes dangerous when it is repetitive without periodic relief to the body.

Good stress fires the body due to naturally-occurring performance enhancing chemicals like adrenalin and cortisol. This heightens ability in the short term and encourages peak performance at such times.

Good stress is sometimes required in individuals to make them achieve peak performance.

Distress on the other hand, when allowed to go unchecked in the longer term, will ultimately decline performance. The constant bombardment by stress-related-chemicals and stimulation will also weaken a person's body, and ultimately, will lead to health's deterioration.

In extreme cases, it can cause psychological problems such as Post Traumatic Stress Disorder or Cumulative Stress Disorder, as it is physically impossible to be anxious and relaxed at the same time.

A **stress event** is a singular or periodic occurrence that can trigger *unusual response* from the body at such times. This may include the death of loved one, the birth of a baby, loss of a job, a divorce, financial loss, etc.

They are sometimes issues of life that are inevitable, oftentimes occurring at unexpected moments. Stress events are sometimes positive, like relocation into a new apartment, change of job, birth of a baby, wedding, etc.

Stress environments on the other hand are concurrent pressures experienced in the course of daily activities.

These environments may include work environment, nature and hazard of job, working conditions, remuneration, existing labor laws, work and family relationships, living environment and neighborhood, largely defined by its conduciveness and ease of access to amenities, ease of commuting, etc.

EFFECT OF STRESS ON MAJOR BODY FUNCTIONS

Normal (relaxed)
Normal rate and blood pressure
Under pressure
Increased rate and blood pressure
Acute pressure
Improved performance
Chronic pressure (stress)
Hypertension and chest pains

Normal (relaxed)
Happy
Under pressure
Serious
Acute pressure
Increased concentration
Chronic pressure (stress)
Anxiety, loss of sense of humor

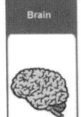

Normal (relaxed)
Blood supply normal
Under pressure
Blood supply up
Acute pressure
Thinks more clearly
Chronic pressure (stress)
Headaches or migraines, tremors

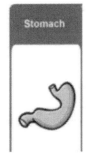

Normal (relaxed)
Normal blood supply and acid secretion
Under pressure
Reduced blood supply and increased acid secretion
Acute pressure
Reduced blood supply reduces digestion
Chronic pressure (stress)
Ulcers due to heartburn & indigestion

EFFECT OF STRESS ON MAJOR BODY FUNCTIONS

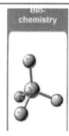

bio-chemistry

Normal (relaxed)
normal: oxygen consumed, glucose
and fats liberated.
Under pressure
oxygen consumption up, glucose
and fats consumption up
Acute pressure
more energy immediately
available
Chronic pressure (stress)
rapid tiredness

Skin

Normal (relaxed)
healthy
Under pressure
decreased blood supply - dry skin
Acute pressure
decreased blood supply
Chronic pressure (stress)
dryness and rashes

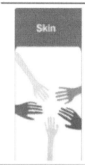

Sexual Organs

Normal (relaxed)
(male) normal. (female) normal periods etc
Under pressure
(m) impotence (decreased blood supply) (f) irregular periods
Acute pressure
decreased blood supply
Chronic pressure (stress)
(m) impotence. (f) menstrual
disorders

Bladder

Normal (relaxed)
Normal
Under pressure
Frequent urination
Acute pressure
Frequent urination due to increased nervous stimulation
Chronic pressure (stress)
Frequent urination, prostatic
symptoms

EFFECT OF STRESS ON MAJOR BODY FUNCTIONS

Bowels

Normal (relaxed)
Normal blood supply and bowel activity
Under pressure
Reduced blood supply and increased bowel activity
Acute pressure
Reduced blood supply reduces digestion
Chronic pressure (stress)
Abdominal pain and

Muscles

Normal (relaxed)
Blood supply normal
Under pressure
Blood supply up
Acute pressure
Improved performance
Chronic pressure (stress)
Muscular tension and pain

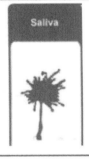

Saliva

Normal (relaxed)
Normal
Under pressure
Reduced
Acute pressure
Reduced
Chronic pressure (stress)
Dry mouth, lump in throat

"The core beverage we need for life and health is water"

- Barry Popkin

CHAPTER TWO
HYDRATION

Water is essential for life.

You can stay only 4 days without water. By weight, our body is about 72% water; another 8% is a combination of chemical compounds and the remaining 20% is bone and solid tissue. Most of the healing and life-giving process that happens in our body happens through Water.

De-hydration is at the root of most diseases. Cancers thrive in de-hydrated environments. A de-hydrated body becomes toxic. Toxicity is the root of most cancers and other life-threatening medical conditions.

The human body is designed to heal itself, if properly supplied with the nutrients to do same. It is amazing how our body components work in synchronicity to bond broken bones, regenerate and replace damaged tissue, attack and destroy hostile organisms. Water plays a vital role in the self–healing process of the body.

The following are some functions of the human body that are largely dependent on water:

a) **Blood** is the vehicle through which nutrients are passed through the body and wastes are conducted for emission from the body. The human blood is made up of about 80% water.

The blood conveys oxygen to needed organs, tissues and cells of the human body. The swiftness of these activities is solely a function of how hydrated the body is at every time. Antibodies are swift and rapid response to invasion by a foreign body. The body mobilizes antibodies to invasion sight through the blood, before the body is ravaged by the invaders. The promptness of the antibodies is also a function of how well hydrated the body is.

b) **Brain** is the human control port where every process in the human body is directed. The human brain is over 80% water. The brain directs activities in the human body by constantly sending and receiving electrical signals through our nervous system. The nervous system is an elaborate system of tiny water ways. The fluid inside our nerves is made up almost completely of water and minerals.

Tiny messengers, called transporter proteins, travel at the speed of light, carrying these life-giving messages to every cell and organ in our body. Like any communication network, the purity of the carrier, our nervous system, affects the speed and clarity of the signal. If the fluid inside of our nerves is laced with traces of chemicals or heavy metals like lead, then the result is a delayed and distorted signal.

It has been well documented that the clarity of these signals has a major effect on our ability to deal with stress and our degree of coordination. Considering the vital role that water plays in our brain and nervous system, its quality is possibly the most basic and essential key to health's longevity.

c) **Energy** generation is vital for the various functions of the human body. The body functions like a complex Hydro Generator, using the elements of nature to become the miracle machine we were intended to be. If the body drops experiences about 5% drop of body fluid, if it loses about 30% of the body's energy, about 30% drop of the body fluid can be fatal.

A large part of our body's energy comes from a compound called ATP, Adenosine-Tri-Phosphate, which is produced during the osmotic flow of water, through the cell membrane, to generate hydroelectric energy. ATP is then stored in energy pools and used as chemical energy in our body.

The mineral content of our body fluids and the absence of contaminants create the proper environment for this natural energy production.

The purity of the water we drink greatly impacts our strength and energy level. Any time a toxic chemical (chlorine included) gets inside our body, we must then use up some of our strength and energy to reduce and repair the damage done by that contaminant.

Water is also what our liver uses to metabolize fat into usable energy. Drinking an abundance of clean chemical-free water speeds up our metabolism and allows our body to assimilate nutrients better, resulting in increased strength and energy

Our water quality is the only part of our personal environment that we can easily obtain total control over. With an abundant intake of clean, healthy water, we allow our body to perform all the healing processes it is naturally capable of.

d) **Detoxification** is the body's method of getting rid of wastes. It is probably the single most important component to optimum health, and the one process that relies most heavily on an adequate intake of clean water.

Our body will use, at least, 8 glasses of water each day, under normal relatively passive activity to maintain the basic bodily functions such as digestion, temperature control, joint lubrication and skin hydration. Each time we exhale, blink our eyes or make any kind of movement at all, we use up some of the available water in our system.

The constant beating of our heart is a water-consuming process. We're continuously depleting the available water level inside our body. In order for our body to properly perform the essential task of filtering and flushing out toxins, we must consume a level of water above the minimum. The more of an excess that exists, the more our body is able to rid itself of the elements that promote disease and aging.

This beautiful and simple process can make a tremendous difference in the degree of health we achieve and maintain, but we have to let it happen by consuming an abundance of clean, healthy water.

Equally important to proper detoxification as quantity, is quality. If we consume water that already contains traces of harsh chemicals, like chlorine or any of the other 2,100 different synthetic chemicals that have already been detected in our water supplies, then such water doesn't have the same ability to pick up and carry out chemical contaminants from our body. Water that is free from contaminants can take on and transport out of our body toxins that find their way into our system through other means.

We are constantly exposed to and ingest a wide variety of harmful chemicals. Everything from the food we eat which contain artificial preservatives, colors and pesticide residue to the clothes we wear, which harbor traces of laundry and dry cleaning chemicals that are absorbed through our skin, all expose us to toxins.

The air we breathe, and virtually everything we touch contains potentially harmful chemicals that are taken in by our body. It is difficult, if not impossible, to maintain the purity of the air we breathe, the things we touch and the food we eat, which only makes the purity of our water even more important.

Healthy Tips for Hydrating Your Body in a Stress Environment

i) Substitute all drinks for water
ii) Abstain from stimulants such as coffee, energy drinks, etc. they de-hydrate your body.
iii) Ensure you have a water bottle which you can carry with you at all time.
iv) Take water mostly at room temperature
v) Take water at regular intervals. It costs nothing to have water-break in the middle of meetings.
vi) Avoid getting de-hydrated at all cost.

"Man is a food-dependent creature. If you don't feed him, he will die. If you feed him improperly, part of him will die."

- Emanuel Cheraskin, MD, DMD (1916-2001

CHAPTER 3
APPROPRIATE FEEDING

Most times, the body's demands for nutrients which are essential for it to perform its critical functions are interpreted as hunger or cravings.

The body does not know food but only understands nutrients.

Feeding the body is essential for the body to carry out its repair work, healing activity, removal of toxins and wastes, replacements of damaged cells with new ones, etc.

The quality of these nutrients is equally important as the quantity at which they are supplied the body for optimal health

Some nutrients are required in large quantity while some are required in trace amounts. Some nutrients can be manufactured by the body while some are not synthesized from within the body.

There are also minerals which the body derives from plants, but not manufactured by plants. Minerals are absorbed from the soil where the plants are planted and are converted to absorbable entity that the body can utilize.

Several factors determine the appropriateness of feeding; such factors include cultivating/farming practices, preservation method, processing method, time of feeding and consistency of feeding.

It should be noted that the following must be considered in labeling any substance as food:

i) It must be close to nature as possible: The introduction of food that has been modified genetically is dangerous to health, and consumption cannot be categorized as appropriate feeding.

ii) It must have been grown organically: Organic farming practices is fast fading away from the world's poorest. The White House of the USA feeds strictly on organic produce. First Lady, Michelle Obama took it a step further by having an organic farm in the White House, responsible for all produce consumed by the America's First family. These are foods with no fertilizers, no chemicals, no growth factors, etc.

iii) It must not be denatured during cooking or processing: Most foods are destroyed during cooking or processing. Rice is polished and the bran removed. The removed bran contains the major nutrients in the rice. What is left in polished rice is nothing compared to what was lost. So much is lost to peeling, boiling, heating and inappropriate washing of food.

While considering appropriate feeding, what to eat is as important as when to eat. The body goes through three stages in 24 hours which sets the body clock for its functions at each stage.

The body goes through the process of Detoxification in the first stage, which starts from 4am and ends by 12noon: this is the period the body is trying to eliminate wastes and end-products of metabolic activities in the body.

This stage requires food that will support the activity of the body for that moment, which is, cleaning of the body. What most people do is to introduce more dirt into the body through what they call food.

This hinders the thorough cleansing of the body as wastes begin to accumulate, creating a toxic environment that's suitable for the growth of diseases and infections.

The second stage is the **assimilation stage** which commences by 12noon and runs till 8:00pm. The body is able to digest ingested substances and better convert them to absorbable forms at this stage as it has carried out self-cleaning in the first stage. Cooked food can be consumed at this stage with some raw foods to aid the assimilation process.

The body goes into repair mode in its third and final stage, which commences by 8pm and runs till 4am the following day. The body begins to replace and repair damaged cells and tissues in the body from the previous day.

Most people load the body with food during these hours, making it difficult for the body to heal itself. Some do not have proper sleep, as this process requires the body to be in a state of rest for optimal repair.

The above divisions play a vital role about when and what we ingest daily.

Individuals who eat to aid the three divisions reduce the pressure on the body systems, making them function at optimum health, while those who continually abuse these three cycles over-burden their systems, reducing their longevity potential.

Busy executives working in stressed conditions can optimize their health by adapting their meal times to the timing of these operations in the body.

A suggested meal plan will be provided at the end of this chapter.

For optimum health for people working in stress environments, incorporating raw foods into their diet is strongly advised.

Why raw foods?

1. Raw foods are easily digested by the body
2. Raw foods still retain most of its nutrients as they have not been damaged via cooking.
3. Raw foods have their digestive enzymes in place, thereby reducing the burden on the digestive system.

4. As we grow, our digestive systems' functions decline, unlike when we are much younger. The ability to digest food like before wanes, especially cooked food.

How to eat raw foods?

1. Smoothies are a blend of a different fruits and vegetables.
2. Juices are extractions from fruits and vegetables
3. Vegetables
4. Salads
5. Plant-based milk like almond milk, rice milk, coconut milk, tiger nut milk, etc.
6. Spices like dill, basil, oregano, ginger, garlic, cinnamon, turmeric, etc.
7. Herbs

Eating should be intentional. People who work in stress environments must choose to eat intentionally, with the primary aim of addressing their health, despite everyday stress.

According to Rev. Tony Akinyemi, "condition-specific eating targets eating to reverse certain ailments and disease conditions in an individual." An example is the elimination of sugary fruits and foods from the diets of individuals with diabetes.

In like manner, people working in stress environments should eat food that will reduce stress on the human body. Such foods that can minimize the stress have a way of controlling the human response to stress and stressors.

A typical breakfast in a stress environment should include the following:

- Breakfast (6am – 10am): Water Melon Juice + Cucumber Juice + Carrot Juice (can be taken at intervals of 2 hours)
  Carrot Juice + Avocado Pear + Apple + Banana(If not Diabetic) (this is a smoothie recipe)
  Ugu Juice + Carrot Juice

  An apple, banana, water melon can be taken between 10 and 11am to prepare the body for lunch.

- Lunch (12 – 3pm)
  Lunch can be any cooked food (provided it does not contain things to avoid)

- Supper (5pm -7pm)
  Most people who work in stress environments do not leave their offices till late. You don't need any cooked food in your system after 7pm.
  It is advisable you feed on raw food for supper. These are fruits and vegetables you can have in your refrigerator in your office and they will nourish your system.

  Salads + raisins (without salad cream)
  Carrot Juice + celery juice + parsely Juice (this will help your nerves rejuvenate and aid your sleeping.

CHAPTER 4
EFFECTIVE REMOVAL OF WASTES

It has been said that there are two root causes of most diseases; toxicity and deficiency.

Each of the trillion cells in our body needs to have an effective means of removing wastes from metabolic products and other toxins triggered by allergic reactions, infections and stress.

Problems arise when wastes are trapped within our systems, without a way of exit. There are several ways the human body removes waste.

Specialized organs perform this function, which keeps the body from harboring toxins which are harmful to human health. The liver is an important organ for removing toxic wastes from the body.

The kidney, lymphatic systems, skin, colon and lungs are all organs for effective removal of toxic wastes from the body.

The DNA also receives counter-instruction from a toxic cell environment. When the cell environment becomes toxic, the DNA goes into survival mode and eventually alters previous and normal codes.

The above alteration is the cause of several cancers in the human body, aptly named according to the location where they are found in the human body.

Another harm toxic materials do when not eliminated from the body is their interference of oxygen transportation to other parts of the body.

Most disease-causing organisms thrive best in oxygen deprived environments, a condition that is occasioned by the presence of toxic products in the cell environment.

In the title "Body Talks", one way of identifying a sickly body is the frequency of bowel movement. The longest duration between the time of ingesting any food substance and the time of fecal expulsion should not be more than 24hours.

Irregular and non-frequent bowel movement can be an initiator of a disease condition in the body.

This process of de-toxification, when absent, can make the body toxic and initiate a disease process. Our diet should aid the body in carrying out its waste elimination function.

As described in the previous chapter, during 4:00am and 12 noon, the body's predominant function is detoxification. The human body can best be aided in this function by ingesting foods that are:

i) High in water content
ii) Raw and loaded with enzymes,
iii) Loaded with the essential minerals, vitamins and other nutritional factors.

Fresh fruit and vegetable juices are foods that fit into this class. Smoothies are also excellent at this time of the day. As earlier described, smoothies are made by blending all kinds of fruit and vegetable juices together in a smoothie maker or a good blender.

For example, tiger nut milk, freshly extracted carrot juice, banana, avocado etc., juices of green vegetables such as celery, spinach, lettuce etc. and a good Omega-3 oil (Udo's oil, flax seed oil, olive oil) can be added.

The consumption of fresh fruit and vegetable juices during the detoxification window (4:00am – 12noon) does not stress the body, as they require minimal energy for digestion.

These foods still contain abundant life-energy that aids digestion when compared to their cooked state which demands much energy for digestion, resulting in exhaustion and fatigue for the individuals after consumption.

The following are ways of putting our body's detoxification in turbo, especially for individuals who work in stress environments:

1. Avoid feeding on cooked food during the detoxification window of each day (4:00am – 12:00pm)
2. Eat mostly fresh fruit and vegetable juices till noon.
3. Drink at least 6 to 8 glasses daily -- preferably water, freshly extracted vegetable juices.
4. Consume cruciferous vegetables like cabbage, broccoli, cauliflower, kale, etc. which supports the liver in removing toxic wastes from the body.

5. Regular moderate exercise helps the skin and lymphatic system eliminates wastes. (This will be dealt with in the subsequent chapter).

6. Saunas also stimulate sweating which aids the skin in the removal of wastes.

*"Today, more than **95% of all chronic disease is caused by** food choice, toxic food ingredients, nutritional deficiencies and lack of physical exercise."*

- Mike Adams, the Health Ranger

"I have always believed that physical exercise is the key; not only to physical fitness, but also peace of mind" **– Nelson Mandela**

CHAPTER 5
OXYGEN AND EXERCISE (AEROBICS)

Renowned biologist, Louis Pasteur coined the word aerobics in the late 19th century, derived from the Greek word *aer* (air) and *bios* (life) - "air life". It was fitness expert, Dr. Kenneth Cooper who later in 1960 coined the word *aerobics* in reference to aerobic exercises that improve cardiovascular conditioning.

When the human body undergoes stress, the body responds by releasing hormones: the chemical by-products of which may be harmful to the body. These by-products are burned off during exercise, reducing stress by releasing endorphins and decreasing fatigue.

Critical is the role played by oxygen in sustaining the human body. Plants take in carbon dioxide and release oxygen, which is critical for human survival. The carbon dioxide helps the plants in their process of manufacturing their food in the presence of sunlight and the green pigment called chlorophyll.

Humans, unlike plants, take in oxygen and require the presence of sunlight with the melanin pigment producing vitamin D3 (among several others), which is needed for the body to absorb mineral nutrients critical for disease prevention and reversal.

The body cell seems to "respire" in a way that it takes in molecular oxygen (as an electron acceptor) and releases carbon dioxide (as an end product), hence, the process is described to be aerobic.

Aerobics starts with proper oxygen circulation, which is why it is important for our homes, offices, gym, etc. to be surrounded with life-giving plants.

Contrary to popular belief, exercise is not just for weight management but for optimal health. The more oxygen gets access into our bodies, the less conducive it is for disease-causing organisms to thrive.

Oxygen aids blood circulation within the body, a vital role needed for survival. During the process of blood circulation, nutrients are distributed throughout the body cells and wastes are carried away from cells for effective elimination from the body.

This effective waste elimination is done through special organs like the liver (which houses about 25% of the blood in the body per time), the kidney (which filters the waste from the blood), colon, lungs (eliminates gaseous waste), the lymphatic system, and the skin (the largest organ in the body).

Hence, the first form of aerobics is proper oxygen exposure before physical exercise is considered. If any of the above organs is deprived of oxygen, the body initiates a disease process. Four minutes is the longest anyone can live without oxygen.

The presence of flowers and plants should be seen as life-givers and not mere aesthetics.

According to Ted Broer, you could lose up to 7% of your muscle mass every 10 years from age 20 unless you exercise regularly. You would have lost about 30% by age 70 due to tissue atrophy.

The muscle mass you lose is replaced by fat tissues. It is a known fact that the body does either of three things to glucose in the human body:

i)   Converts to fuel (ATP) and use it up immediately
ii)   Converts and store up as a reserve energy
iii) Converts and store up as fats in adipose tissue

While protein can be converted to glucose, unfortunately fats cannot be reversed through conversion back into glucose (a form usable by the body) but can only be burned up through exercise.

According to Ted Broer, the functions of the human body are regulated by hormones, while your hormones are regulated by the basal metabolic rate.

The thyroid hormone regulates metabolism within the human body. The pancreas secrete insulin and according to Ted Broer, glucagon.

Fats are accumulated in an orderly way in the human body starting from the stomach, waist line, arms, etc. They also leave in that order, starting from the last and ending with the first.

This account for the longer time it takes to burn belly fats. It takes an hour work-out to burn 100 calories but a meal high in glycemic index will restore the fats.

Exercise aids the detoxification process in the body as circulation becomes effective; wastes are eliminated promptly to prevent toxicity which can create a conducive environment for initiating a disease condition.

Circulation in the body is carried out by the blood and the lymph. The blood is mobilized through pumping by the heart while the lymph is mobilized through physical exercise.

Many tissues depend on the lymph to provide nutrients and carry away wastes. If the lymph does not circulate, then the tissues suffocate in their own acidic waste products.

Cardiovascular exercises put the heart, lungs and the network of blood vessels, veins and capillaries in turbo. This enables the body release glucagon from the pancreas especially when the exercise is carried out on an empty stomach in the morning.

The glucagon released will speed up the burning of the fat for fuel. Cardiovascular exercise, like any other exercise, should be done with due consultation with your health care provider.

Exercise also plays the role of keeping our muskulo-skeletal health at its peak as we age. Bone mineralization is initiated through weight-bearing or strength-training exercise. This prevents osteoporosis in adult's life.

E.R. Eichner stated that "After exercise bouts lasting longer than 30minutes, the number of white blood cells may be elevated for 24hours or more before returning to normal levels" – (*Infection, Immunity, and Exercise: What to tell patients" Physician and Sports Medicine, January 1993, 125-135).*

Exercise raises the immunity level of the human body, placing the body soldiers on high alert to fight enemy invasion.

With all the functions stating the importance of helping our body utilize oxygen through fitness exercises, it shows whoever is not *intentionally* engaged in fitness activities is setting their body up for diseases.

Dr. Paul C. Reisser describes four reasons people don't engage in physical fitness activities.

i) Motivation: Until you determine what is in it for you, you may never be well motivated to go through the process. Many jobs are very unattractive but the pay keeps the worker motivated enough to wake up each morning and report for duty. Writing down what you intend to achieve and setting them before you as goals will help motivate you.

ii) Schedule: People working in stress environments often wish for an extension to the 24-hour daily time allocation. A few things determine how well you will live and how long you will enjoy the wealth you are struggling to make: exercise is one. Your life depends on it.

Sedentary living is most common among working class elites, a condition giving rise to the prevalence of several terminal ailments in recent times.

iii) Creativity: There are several activities that can help to actively move your muscles while keeping a busy schedule. There are a few activities you need to take away from your delegation list to help extend your life. You may have to figure out such activities to cure the time constraint and enjoy the process.

iv) Self-discipline: The greatest hindrance to health is indulgence, weak self-will and self-discipline. Many people just resign to fate and do nothing to improve their health. This is different from the occasional non-desire to hit the gym; this happens many times but can be overcome through peer/group motivation. Having someone around you to exercise with will help you during those moments.

The following is a suggested aerobics planning for individuals in stress environments:

1. Surround yourself with green plants that have good exposure to sunlight.

2. Consult your health care giver before commencing any exercise program.

3. Engage in stretch exercise first to allow your muscles adjust as you probably might not have done this since high school. You can stretch first thing in the morning by raising your hands high, bending gradually and touching your toes. You can do this for a few days before going on to another form of exercise.

4. You can engage in cardiovascular exercise like brisk walking for about 30 minutes. (If you want to lose weight, do this on an empty stomach with only water intake).

5. "Skip the elevator" – if you work in buildings with several floors, you can start by climbing down the stairs or skip the elevator for a few floors and join the elevator on higher floors, to complete your movement within the building. Graduate from skipping the elevator for a few floors to completely climbing the stairs at least once daily. It is called stair walking.

6. Strength training can be done by engaging the use of dumb bells. You can have them around your office, in your car, while not driving or at home.

7. Jumping rope for 15 minutes

8. Shooting baskets (basketball) for 30 minutes*

9. Taking water moderately, especially clean and mineralized water.

10. Dancing fast for 30 minutes

11. Bicycling 4 miles in 15 minutes

12. Swimming is a great exercise that combines cardiovascular, stretching and strength exercise in one. You can get away with an hour swimming in a week for optimal health.

You can initiate a fitness group in your workplace where people are encouraged to work-out in the work place. Exercising with a partner helps you achieve your exercise goals while you can encourage each other when boredom and fatigue sets in.

It is also important to be careful of the environment during exercise. Roads and routes must be such that guarantee the safety of users.

Work-out with a partner helps you achieve your exercise goals while you can encourage each other when boredom and fatigue set in.

To prevent injuries, fatigue and loss of motivation, the commencement and changes in exercise must be gradual. It is advisable to stop exercise immediately you feel any pain in the chest. You may have to consult your doctor immediately if the pain persists for a few minutes.

Your pulse is a guide to pace your exercise. Your health care provider should guide you on this.

It is important that everyone with a very busy schedule should attempt to accumulate about 30 minutes of moderate-intense physical activity daily.

It is not compulsory for the 30 minutes to be at a stretch, but can be done through two 15 minutes or three 10 minutes.

*"The best six doctors anywhere that no one can deny are **SUNSHINE**, rest, exercise, air, diet and exercise"*

– Wayne Fields

CHAPTER 6
EXPOSURE TO SUNLIGHT

Sunlight is one of God's several provisions to sustain life on planet earth. Plants depend on sunlight to manufacture their food with the aid of their green pigmentation and the presence of carbon dioxide.

Recent researches have shown the importance of sunlight in the production of Vitamin D, also labeled as the "sunshine vitamin".

Vitamin D is produced by the skin's response to UV radiation, primarily through sun exposure, which affects 10 percent of the genes in the human body.

The importance of Vitamin D in health and wellness is as the importance of Sunlight to plants in the production of their foods for survival.

Sunlight is abundant in nature except for people in the arctic regions. However, several people are deficient in Vitamin D because of the way they have chosen to relate with exposure to sunlight.

Over-exposure to sunlight causes skin cancer. Appropriate exposure is also a relative term and differs from an individual to another, largely because of skin color and time of exposure.

Dark skin requires about five to six times more solar exposure than pale skin, for equivalent vitamin D photosynthesis

Studies have linked vitamin D, known as the "sunshine vitamin," to protection against colon, kidney, and breast cancer. It's also linked to improvements in bone health and overall mortality.

Neurological, cardiovascular, and immune diseases are associated with vitamin D deficiency. By increasing your exposure to sunlight, you can decrease your risk for these diseases.

Vitamin D combined with other cancer treatments also tends to improve the patient's prognosis. However, dietary, genetic, and environmental factors can mask the effects of vitamin D on the body.

Sunlight shuts off the body's production of melatonin, a hormone produced at night that makes you feel drowsy. Constant exposure to sunlight can help your body maintain its circadian rhythm. Your circadian rhythm is a 24-hour cycle that regulates biochemical, physiological, and behavioral processes and makes you feel tired when it's dark outside.

When people are exposed to sunlight or very bright artificial light in the morning, their nocturnal melatonin production occurs sooner, and they enter into sleep more easily at night.

Melatonin production also shows a seasonal variation relative to the availability of light, with the hormone produced for a longer period in the winter than in the summer. The melatonin rhythm phase advancement caused by exposure to bright morning light has been effective against insomnia, premenstrual syndrome, and seasonal affective disorder (SAD).

As diurnal creatures, we humans are programmed to be outdoors while the sun is shining and home in bed at night.

This is why melatonin is produced during the dark hours and stops upon optic exposure to daylight. This pineal hormone is a key pacesetter for many of the body's circadian rhythms.

Going outside for 15 minutes at the same time every day, preferably in the morning, tells your body that it's no longer nighttime. Sunlight that's unhindered by sunglasses will reach the brain's pineal gland more easily and signal it to stop releasing melatonin.

Researchers from the Baker Heart Research Institute in Melbourne found that levels of serotonin—a neurotransmitter that regulates appetite, sleep, memory, and mood—are lower during the winter than the summer.

The research team noted that the only factor that affected participants' moods was the amount of sunlight they were exposed to on any given day. More sunlight meant better moods; less sunlight led to symptoms of depression.

The melatonin precursor, serotonin, is also affected by exposure to daylight. Normally produced during the day, serotonin is only converted to melatonin in darkness. Serotonin plays an important role in weight management especially for people with uncontrollable appetite.

Vitamin D deficiencies have been associated to higher visceral fat production, which leads to obesity and subsequent health-threatening diseases, including diabetes and cardiovascular issues.

According to Dr. Micheal Holicks, "obesity is associated with vitamin D deficiency. The reason is that the vitamin D is trapped within the fat and cannot easily exit. As a result, obese patients need at least twice as much vitamin D as a normal weighted individual, in order to maintain a normal vitamin D status".

The study suggests that low levels of serotonin directly correlate with seasonal affective disorder, which most often occurs during winter months. Individuals with eating disorder are usually plagued with depression and often use food as mood lightener.

Moderately high serotonin levels result in more positive moods and calm yet focused mental outlook. Indeed, SAD has been linked with low serotonin levels during the day as well as with a phase delay in nighttime melatonin production.

It was recently found that mammalian skin can produce serotonin and transform it into melatonin, and that many types of skin cells express receptors for both serotonin and melatonin.

Vitamin D enhances calcium and phosphorus absorption, controlling the flow of calcium into and out of bones to regulate bone-calcium metabolism.

Dr. Michael Holick, a medical professor and director of the Bone Health Care Clinic at Boston University Medical Center, says, "The primary physiologic function of vitamin D is to maintain serum calcium and phosphorous levels within the normal physiologic range to support most metabolic functions, neuromuscular transmission, and bone mineralization."

Without sufficient vitamin D, bones will not form properly. In children, this causes rickets, a disease characterized by growth retardation and various skeletal deformities, including the hallmark bowed legs.

A Swedish epidemiologic study published in the December 2006 issue of *Diabetologia* found that sufficient vitamin D status in early life was associated with a lower risk of developing type-1 diabetes.

Non-obese mice of a strain predisposed to develop type 1 diabetes showed an 80% reduced risk of developing the disease when they received a daily dietary dose of 1,25(OH)D, according to research published in the June 1994 issue of the same journal.

A Finnish study published on the 3rd of November, 2001 in *The Lancet,* showed that children who received 2,000 IU vitamin D per day from 1 year of age on had an 80% decreased risk of developing type 1 diabetes later in life, whereas children who were vitamin D deficient had a fourfold increased risk.

There is also a connection with metabolic syndrome, a cluster of conditions that increases one's risk for Type-2 diabetes and cardiovascular disease.

A study in the September 2006 issue of *Progress in Biophysics and Molecular Biology* demonstrated that in young and elderly adults, serum 25(OH)D was inversely correlated with blood glucose concentrations and insulin resistance.

Some studies have demonstrated high prevalence of low vitamin D levels in people with type 2 diabetes, although it is not clear whether this is a cause of the disease or an effect of another causative factor—for example, lower levels of physical activity (in this case, outdoor activity in particular).

The sun's rays lower blood pressure as exposure significantly lowers blood pressure in individuals with high blood pressure. On the other hand, pharmaceutical drugs such as Statins have side effects, such as robbing the body of Coenzyme Q10. CoQ10 is essential for cellular and heart energy.

Sunlight penetrates deep into the skin to cleanse the blood and blood vessels. Medical literature published in Europe showed that people with atherosclerosis (hardened arteries) improved with sun exposure.

Sunlight increases oxygen content in human blood. And, it also enhances the body's capacity to deliver oxygen to the tissues; very similar to the effects of exercise.

In Summary, Vitamin D in the body, is essential for many functions such as:

- bone health
- anti-cancer
- supports the immune system
- protects against dementia and brain aging
- good for loosing excess fat and weight management

- essential for decreasing symptoms of asthma
- strengthens teeth and bone in children
- calcium and phosphorus absorption

The following are suggestions for individuals working in stress environments on how to get optimal exposure to sunlight

i. You need the early sunshine which comes between 7 and 8:30 in the morning. Try to get about 15 minutes exposure daily. You can do this while in your car driving (ensure the windows are down as the UV radiation can be screened by the car's window glass).

ii. For people in jobs in which sunlight exposure is limited, full-spectrum lighting may be helpful.

iii. Sunglasses may further limit the eyes' access to full sunlight, thereby altering melatonin rhythms. Going shades-free in the daylight, even for just 10–15 minutes, could confer significant health benefits.

iv. Vitamin D3 supplements are also available and you can use daily according to your body requirements.

Caution:

According to Dr. Joseph Mercola, "While sun exposure is your best source for vitamin D, it's important to understand that *not all sun exposure will allow for vitamin D production*."

Sunlight is composed of about 1,500 wavelengths, but the only wavelength that makes your body produce vitamin D are UVB-rays, when they hit exposed skin. The UVB-rays from the sun must pass through the atmosphere and reach where you are on the earth in order for this to take place.

Most people know that D2 – the synthetic version commonly prescribed by doctors – is not as potent as D3. Each microgram of orally consumed 25-hydroxyvitamin D3 is about five times more effective in raising serum 25(OH)D than an equivalent amount of vitamin D2.

However, besides being less potent, D2 supplements may actually do more harm than good overall.

*Two causes have been advanced as the major causes of all illnesses and diseases. **Deficiency,** which is the absence or shortage of critical nutrient factors for growth and general well-being, and **Toxicity,** which is the presence of substances harmful to the human body.*

CHAPTER 7
DIETARY SUPPLEMENTS

Normally, you should be able to get all the nutrients you need from a balanced diet. However, taking supplements can provide additional nutrients when your diet is lacking or when certain health conditions cause you to develop an insufficiency or deficiency.

So much is being advertised and marketed regarding supplements to the disadvantage of the uninformed consumer.

Several phrases like "lose weight", "burn fat", "improve performance", "magic formula", "cures all" etc. are being used to rip unsuspecting buyers in the name of dietary supplementation.

According to the US Food and Drug Administration "Dietary supplements include vitamins, minerals, and other less familiar substances — such as herbals, botanicals, amino acids, enzymes, and animal extracts. Dietary supplements are also marketed in forms such as tablets, capsules, softgels, and gelcaps."

Supplements become necessary because:

i. Modern farming methods deplete soils, which means insufficient mineral content to produce nutrient dense vegetables and fruit.

ii. Long transit times for some foods, which decreases nutrient quality, and

iii. Cooking methods of cooked foods encourage the loss of vitamins, minerals, antioxidants, and enzymes.

According to Kathleen M. Zeeman, MPH, RD in her title "What Supplements Can and Can't Do", it is very important to note the following:

1. Supplements are not meant to be a substitute for food

   Vitamins and other dietary supplements are not intended to be a food substitute. They cannot replace all of the nutrients and benefits of whole foods.

   "They can plug nutrition gaps in your diet, but it is short-sighted to think your vitamin or mineral is the ticket to good health -- the big power is on the plate, not in a pill," explains Roberta Anding, MS, RD, a spokesperson for the American Dietetic Association and director of sports nutrition at Texas Children's Hospital in Houston.

2. Any supplement marketed as a whole/only, quick fix, one-size-fits-all remedy is wrong marketing

   If it sounds too good to be true, it probably is. It is unlikely that a vitamin or mineral can deliver on a promise like helping you lose weight. A promise like that goes beyond the function of a supplement.

"Don't expect a vitamin or mineral to do anything more than it does in food", says Anding.

An overall healthy diet, appropriate lifestyle and regular physical activity remains the holistic option to prevent chronic disease, not supplements.

Two causes have been advanced as the major causes of all illnesses and diseases: *Deficiency,* which is the absence or shortage of critical nutrient factors for growth and general well-being and *Toxicity,* which is the presence of substances harmful to the human body.

Addressing the two above mentioned causes will guarantee super health for anyone.

According to Dr. Joel Wallach and Dr. Ma Lan in their book "Dead Doctors Don't Lie", about 90 nutrients (some essential and some non-essential) have been discovered to be required for the human body. The deficiency of one of these 90 nutrients can be responsible for a minimum of 10 health conditions.

Supplementing arises to address the deficiency that may occur due to reasons earlier stated. There are severe consequences of deficiency in the human body. Some of these are:

i)   Deficiency of folic acid in women of reproductive age can lead to birth defects. Most common is *spina bifida* which is a defective development of the spinal cord in babies whose mothers are deficient in folic acid before and during pregnancy.

ii) Selenium deficiency can lead to anemia, infertility, liver cirrhosis, cancer, etc.

iii) Zinc deficiency can also lead to infertility in men, causing low sperm count, body odor, low sense of smell and taste, anemia, heart defects, palpitations, congenital defects in babies whose mothers were deficient before and during pregnancy, etc.

iv) According to Dr. Joel Wallach in his book "Dead Doctors Don't Lie", copper deficiency in human beings present itself first as white, gray or silver hair. Copper is required to manufacture hair pigment for blood, red, brown or black hair, says Dr. Wallach.

Copper deficiency can also cause skin wrinkles, spider veins, varicose veins, hemorrhoids, iron storage diseases, and iron resistant anemia, violent behavior, blind rage, learning disabilities in children, cerebral palsy, etc.

v) Manganese deficiency can lead to deafness, asthma, convulsions, infertility, still births, loss of libido in male, retarded growth rate, etc.

vi) Magnesium deficiency can cause asthma, anorexia, growth failure, menstrual migraines, depression, tremors, vertigo, etc.

vii)   Iodine is a mineral with critical functions in the human body as it relates with the thyroid. Its deficiency can lead to hypothyroidism with symptoms like fatigue, cold intolerance, low sex drive, excessive weight gain, elevated blood cholesterol, dry skin and hair, poor memory, goiter, etc.

Its deficiency can also lead to hypothyroidism with symptoms such as insomnia, heart intolerance, rapid pulse, excessive sweating, heat intolerance, weight loss, goiter, increased appetite, irritability, nervousness, etc.

viii)   Chromium deficiency can lead to low blood sugar, prediabetes, type II diabetes, ADD/ADHD, depression, hyperactivity, panic attacks, impaired growth, infertility, decreased sperm count, elevated blood cholesterol, etc.

ix)   Calcium deficiency results in osteoporosis, dowager's hump, lordosis, receding gums, osteomalacia, degenerate arthritis, hypertension, insomnia, kidney stones, PMS, low back pain, osteofibrosis, prolonged clotting time, etc.

The use of supplements is of great importance to individuals working in stress environments. As stressed earlier in this chapter, it should not be an alternative to healthy diet, lifestyle and physical activity.

"Temperance is moderation in the things that are good and total abstinence from the things that are foul."

---Frances E. Willard

CHAPTER 8
ABSTINENCE AND MODERATION

Toxicity has been addressed as the other cause of diseases which we have defined as the presence of harmful substances, metabolic wastes, toxins, etc. in the human body.

As much as getting rid of these substances is important to the human body, restricting their access to the human body is fundamental to healthy living.

Abstinence and moderation come to play as all efforts must be employed to restrict the access and production of toxic substances while those that cannot be restricted must be eliminated from the body within stipulated time.

The following are what we are expected to abstain from, especially for individuals with major health conditions:

1. Common Salt (refined salt)
    i)   Common salt or refined salt should be completely eliminated, especially in individuals above the age of 40.
    ii)   Most commercial-refined salts have been harvested mechanically from various salt mines as brine. Brine is a highly concentrated solution of water and salt. Prior to mechanical evaporation, the brine is often treated with chemicals (sulfuric acid and chlorine) to remove impurities including healthy minerals and elements.
    iii)   Refined salt may contain anti-caking, free flowing, or conditioning agents. These agents may include

sodium ferrocyanide, ammonium citrate, and aluminum silicate. None of these products have any positive effects in the body

   iv) Use Himalayan Crystal Salt or Sea Salt moderately in your cooking.
   v) Unrefined salt is packed with essential minerals and supplies the body with a proper balance of sodium and chloride with over 80 trace minerals.
   vi) Never add salt to an already prepared food.

2. White Flour Products:
   i) White flour products include white bread, cake, donut, meat-pie, noodles, biscuits, pancake, pasta, chin-chin, buns, etc. made from white flour.
   ii) The wheat grain, also called the kernel or wheat berry, consists of three components; bran (source of dietary fiber), wheat germ (rich in vitamins and contains unsaturated fats) and the endosperm (the starchy, soft and white 85% portion of the kernel)
   iii) When machines pulverize kernels into flour, even whole-grain flour, what's left behind is a starchy powder capable of wreaking havoc on the body.
   iv) Whole-grain wheat contains the entire component of the grain, while white flour has only the endosperm, which includes gluten without the vitamins, minerals and fiber.
   v) Consuming white flour can lead to a number of problems in the body, including blood-sugar blues, cardiovascular diseases, diabetes, cancer, etc.
   vi) Eat whole-grain bread, whole oats, buck wheat, quinoa, whole cornmeal or their combination in a multi grain product.

vii)   Buy cereals that are also made from whole grains.

viii) Always look out for pasta made from whole grain.

3. Hydrogenated and partially hydrogenated fats

i) This includes margarine, lard, shortening, etc.

ii) Poly-unsaturated fatty acids that occur naturally in food are in the *cis* form, while the process of extracting or processing oils from plants or seeds and the process of creating partially hydrogenated products from them generate a significant proportion of *trans* fatty acids.

iii) *Trans* fatty acids raise LDL cholesterol (the bad type of cholesterol) and triglyceride levels.

iv) The Food and Drug Administration (FDA) in 2009 estimated that the amount of *trans* fatty acids resulting from food labeling as well as voluntary efforts by manufacturers to reduce the amounts of these compounds in foods will prevent 600 to 1,200 heart attacks and save 250 to 500 lives yearly)

v) Organic unsalted butter can be used moderately.

4. Fried foods and junk foods

i) These include all refined, processed, canned and polished foods, polished white rice, etc.

ii) Frying has been implicated in the production of acryl amide in certain foods like potatoes.

iii) Acryl amide has been found to be a carcinogen in cancer studies and experiments conducted on rats. The compound is created when a sugar and an amino acid called 'asparagines' combine during high-temperature cooking or heating for extended lengths of time.

iv) Frying also denatures the structure of the oil we use by converting them to trans-fat.

v) Cholesterol produced with trans-fat will have reduced permeability which will restrict the entrance of nutrients into the cell and the exit of waste products from the cell, making the cell nutrient deficient and the cell environment toxic as it will not be effective in waste elimination, making the cell suitable for cancer development.

vi) It also affects enzymatic procedures in the body, resulting in conditions such as slow digestion.

vii) Eat brown rice or *Ofada Rice*.

5. Sugar, Aspartame, Saccharin, Artificial Sweeteners:

i) Aspartame and refined sugar are twin devils. Aspartame is found in no-sugar/sugar-free products and drinks.

ii) Aspartame is used largely in the energy-drink industry. One major component of aspartame is formaldehyde used in embalming dead bodies in the mortuary.

iii) According to Dr. Joseph Marcola, Aspartame, a sweetener used in the food industry in place of sugar has been found in the production of energy drinks, sugar-free drinks, chewable vitamin C, flavored drinks, etc. and is by far the most dangerous item in the market that is added to foods.

    iv)   Overwhelming evidence proves that, it actually promotes weight gain, and is linked to a higher risk of diabetes, headaches, vision problems, high blood pressure, and heart diseases. Aspartame intake is a worse evil when compared with sugar consumption.

    v)   As explained by Dr. Rusell Blaylock, sugar has a profound influence on the brain function, and enhances your psychological function.

    vi)   When consumed in excess amounts, the body releases excess amounts of insulin, which in turn causes a drop in your blood sugar, also known as hypoglycemia. Hypoglycemia in turn causes your brain to secrete glutamate.

    vii)   Use Stevia, Therasweet, Agave Nectar, Maple Syrup, etc. Stevia is particularly good for DIABETICS.

    viii)   Make your own drinks freshly extracted and unpasteurized juices)

6. Alcoholic beverages, tobacco, hard drugs, Caffeine-containing substances – coffee, black tea, cocoa products, etc.

    i)   Caffeine tolerance varies between individuals.

    ii)   Caffeine has been known to be addictive and is at the root of several medical conditions.

    iii)   Caffeine is also known to cause agitation and restlessness in young people.

    iv)   Cola drinks (contain caffeine) is also implicated in unstable behavior in kids.

    v)   According to The Mayo Clinic, dizziness, irritability, increased urination, increased blood pressure, heart palpitations, nausea etc. can all develop at an intolerable dosage on caffeine.

vi) Drink green Tea, camomile, nettle, raspberry Tea, Mint Tea, Hibiscus Tea, fennel tea, etc.

vii) Carob tea is a good substitute for the various cocoa products grown on GMOs.

7. COW MILK & DIARY PRODUCTS:

i) This includes liquid milk, pasteurized milk, powdered milk, skimmed milk, condensed milk, ice-cream etc.,

ii) Human beings are the only mammals that feed on milk after being weaned from breast milk which is not necessary

iii) Cow milk has been seriously compromised for commercial reasons with growth hormones and other substances which may inhibit the absorption of calcium and other minerals in children

iv) Hormone alteration is an underlying cause of several disease conditions. Hormone alteration can be triggered by the growth factor in cows used in commercial production of cow-based milk.

v) Commercial farmers sometimes raise these cows on antibiotics which still find its way into the milk consumed in all its form.

vi) According to Dr. Linda Folden Palmer, D.C. of the Natural Child Project, dairy's high calcium causes relative deficiencies in magnesium and other bone-building minerals, and its high phosphorus and animal protein reduces calcium availability. Don't be deceived by the adverts/commercials.

vii) Use plant-derived milk, except soya milk. Use almond milk, coconut milk, oat milk, tiger-nut milk, etc.

8. Animal Products: especially red meat, imported poultry products, pork products, dairy products, etc.
9. MSG (Monosodium Glutamate)
    i)   This includes packaged seasonings, cubed seasonings, seasonings for noodles, and all other chemical seasonings, etc.
    ii)   Monosodium Glutamate is not a nutrient but a chemical that is also known as an exotoxin.
    iii) Mono-Sodium Glutamate (MSG) over-stimulates the cells, leading to cell-death and it has been implicated as a leading cause of cancer and hormonal imbalance in individuals over the years.
    iv)   According to Dr. Joseph Mercola, glutamate is a "messenger molecule" that serves an important function in your body. However, when excess amounts of glutamate are excreted, it can wreak havoc with your brain and nervous system, causing a variety of side effects such as agitation, depression, anger, anxiety and panic attacks.
    v)   Use Herbal Seasonings such as Curry Powder, Thyme, Basil, Oregano, Dill, *Iru, Ogiri, Dawadawa*, cinnamon, etc.

"A smile will gain you more ten years of life"

– Chinese Proverb

CHAPTER 9
LAUGHTER THERAPY

Have you ever wondered why the poor who work in bus parks and garages are always happy and in an excited mood all day, while a well-paid executive is depressed despite the good things of life he enjoys?

He who laughs, lasts! — *Mary Pettibone Poole*

According to Melinda Smith, M.A and Jeanne Seagal Ph.D. of the Harvard Health, laughter is good for your health as:

i) Laughter relaxes the whole body. A good, hearty laugh relieves physical tension and stress, leaving your muscles relaxed for up to 45 minutes after.

ii) Laughter boosts the immune system. Laughter decreases stress hormones and increases immune cells and infection-fighting antibodies, thus improving your resistance to disease.

iii) Laughter triggers the release of endorphins which is the body's natural feel-good chemicals. Endorphins promote an overall sense of well-being and can even temporarily relieve pain.

iv) Laughter protects the heart. Laughter improves the function of blood vessels and increases blood flow, which can help protect you against a heart attack and other cardiovascular problems.

Physical Health Benefits of Laughter
i) Boosts immunity
ii) Lowers stress hormones

iii) Decreases pain
iv) Relaxes your muscles
v) Prevents heart disease

Mental Health Benefits of laughter:
i) Adds joy and zest to life
ii) Eases anxiety and fear
iii) Relieves stress
iv) Improves mood
v) Enhances resilience

Social Benefits of laughter:
i) Strengthens relationships
ii) Attracts others to us
iii) Enhances teamwork
iv) Helps defuse conflict
v) Promotes group bonding

The link between laughter and mental health
i) Laughter dissolves distressing emotions. You can't feel anxious, angry, or sad when you're laughing.
ii) Laughter helps you relax and recharge. It reduces stress and increases energy, enabling you to stay focused and accomplish more.
iii) Humor shifts perspective, allowing you to see situations in a more realistic, less threatening light. A humorous perspective creates psychological distance, which can help you avoid feeling overwhelmed.

According to Harvard Health, here are some ways to start:
i) Smile. Smiling is the beginning of laughter. Like laughter, it's contagious. Pioneers in "laugh therapy," find that it's possible to laugh without even experiencing a funny

event. The same holds for smiling. When you look at someone or see something even mildly pleasing, practice smiling.

ii) Count your blessings. Literally make a list. The simple act of considering the good things in your life will distance you from negative thoughts that are a barrier to humor and laughter. When you're in a state of sadness, you have further to travel to get to humor and laughter.

iii) When you hear laughter, move toward it. Sometimes humor and laughter are private, a shared joke among a small group, but usually not. More often, people are very happy to share something funny because it gives them an opportunity to laugh again and feed off the humor you find in it. When you hear laughter, seek it out and ask, "What's funny?"

iv) Spend time with fun, playful people. These are people who laugh easily—both at themselves and at life's absurdities—and who routinely find the humor in everyday events. Their playful point of view and laughter are contagious.

v) Bring humor into conversations. Ask people, "What's the funniest thing that happened to you today? This week? In your life?"

Laughter is the "Best Medicine" for Your Heart, describes a study that found that laughter helps to prevent heart disease. (University of Maryland Medical Center)

One essential characteristic that helps us laugh is not taking ourselves too seriously.

Some events are clearly sad and not occasions for laughter. But most events in life don't carry an overwhelming sense of either sadness *or* delight. They fall into the gray zone of ordinary life—giving you the choice to laugh or not.

Ways to help yourself see the lighter side of life:

i)   Laugh at yourself. Share your embarrassing moments. The best way to take yourself less seriously is to talk about times when you took yourself too seriously.

ii) Attempt to laugh at situations rather than bemoan them. Look for the humor in a bad situation, and uncover the irony and absurdity of life. This will help improve your mood and the mood of those around you.

iii) Surround yourself with reminders to lighten up. Keep a toy on your desk or in your car. Put up a funny poster in your office. Choose a computer screensaver that makes you laugh. Frame photos of you and your family or friends having fun.

iv) Keep things in perspective. Many things in life are beyond your control—particularly the behavior of other people. While you might think taking the weight of the world on your shoulders is admirable, on the long run, it's unrealistic, unproductive, unhealthy, and even egotistical.

v)   Deal with your stress. Stress is a major impediment to humor and laughter.

vi) Pay attention to children and emulate them. They are the experts in playing, taking life lightly, and laughing.

CHAPTER 10
REGULAR MEDICAL CHECK-UP

After disease prevention, the next important pro-activity to stay alive and healthy is early detection.

Especially for individuals crossing the 40s, routine medical check-up is critical as various diseases and illnesses tend to show up in latter life.

Every day, we are stressed out and usually spend long working hours in the office to finance our kid's education and pay for bills. Regular medical check-up has become very essential to enable the individual to detect his actual state of health and any disease that he may be carrying at an early stage and better still prevent illness occurring in the first place. Some tests save so many lives that it is definitely worth the money spent on it

Not all serious medical problems have symptoms in their early stages. A physical exam could detect something while it is still treatable or while the diagnosis is still favorable. If you maintain a routine of regular checkups, you greatly reduce the chances of getting sick in the first place.

The object of staying healthy should be in identifying symptoms before they become incurable. There are several options of medical checkups like Basic, General, and Comprehensive and so on.

Regular check-ups enable us to take remedial action in time. But actually a large number of people think it is foolish and a waste of time and money.

If a person develops cancer, he or she can improve the chance that it will be detected early with regular medical check-ups and regular self-examinations. Often, a doctor can find early cancer during a physical exam or during routine tests, even if the person has no symptoms

According to the Centre for Disease Control (CDC), regular health exams and tests can help find problems before they start. They also can help find problems early, when your chances for treatment and cure are better.

Nearly half of the health disorders we are facing today are somehow connected to our stress. Due to the economic conditions being felt by families, there has been a sharp increase in stress-related health disorders, which in some cases, are life-threatening.

Because of the increasing hypertension symptoms, many of us, instead of visiting the doctor for cold, flu or constant stomach ache are now dealing with these illnesses through some form of home remedies.

Through home remedies, one can deal with the symptoms of these health issues for the time being, but the real cause of these problems remain unaddressed and results in a complicated disease in the future, except during routine medical exam.

Experts suggest that everybody should see doctors regularly, regardless of age, sex and health. Even if you are enjoying good health, visit your doctor once or twice a year for a thorough checkup and medical advice. Seeing a doctor is something that each and every person owes themselves and the family that they love.

You can safeguard and enhance your health, perhaps for many decades, by having certain screening tests a few times in your 20s.

The tests are used for early detection of some of the more common and potentially serious diseases occurring in adults, such as sexually transmitted diseases, cancers, diabetes, and heart disease.

Screening tests can find certain conditions in their earliest and most treatable stages, even before you notice symptoms. With information from screening tests, your health care provider can work with you to develop preventive measures that will help you remain healthier in your later years.

For example, a routine cholesterol test could reveal your risk of developing heart disease, allowing you to take preventive measures—like lifestyle changes—before you develop a serious condition.

According to *The Massachusetts Health Quality Partners*, the following periodic health evaluation is important at every age:

I.   Obtain initial/interval medical history
II.   Perform age-appropriate physical exam.
III. Engage preventive screenings and counseling.
IV.   Update immunizations where necessary.

Frequency

18-29 Years	30-39 Years	40-49 Years	50-64 Years	65+ Years
Annually for ages 18-21. Every 1-3 years, depending on risk factors, for ages 22-29.	Every 1-3 years, depending on risk factors.	Every 1-3 years, depending on risk factors.	Annually	Annually

The following are a list of lab screenings appropriate for different age groups:

LABS AND CANCER SCREENINGS

Breast Cancer

18-39 Years	40-49 Years	50-64 Years	65+ Years
Starting at age 20, perform clinical breast exam at all periodic health evaluations and counsel on the benefits and limitations of self-exams. Advise mammography or other imaging test for patients at high risk. Risk factors include: family history of premenopausal breast cancer (mother or sister) and personal history of breast/ovarian/ endometrial cancer.	Perform clinical breast exam and counsel on the benefits and limitations of self-exams. Discuss the benefits and risks of biennial mammography with patient. Decision to conduct screening at discretion of clinician/patient based on risk factors and patient values regarding benefits/harms.	Perform clinical breast exam and counsel on the benefits and limitations of self-exams. Conduct mammography every two years or more frequently at discretion of clinician/patient based on risk factors and patient values regarding benefits/harms.	Perform clinical breast exam and counsel on the benefits and limitations of self-exams. Conduct mammography every two years through age 74 or more frequently at clinician/patient discretion based on risk factors and patient values regarding benefits harms. After age 75 discuss benefits and limitations in relation to co-morbidity based on patient's health status.

Cervical Cancer

21-29 Years	30-65+ Years
Initiate Pap test and pelvic exam at age 21, or earlier at physician/patient discretion. Perform Pap test and pelvic exam every three years through age 29.	Perform pelvic exam and Pap test every 1-3 years, depending on risk factors. Risk factors include: failure to receive regular Pap tests; history of cervical tumors; infection with HPV (human papillomavirus) or other sexually transmitted diseases; high-risk sexual behavior; and HIV/AIDS. After age 30, physician/patient can discuss screening with combination of cytology and human papillomavirus (HPV) testing every 5 years. Omit Pap test if a woman has had a hysterectomy for benign disease, or after age 65 if there is documented evidence of consistently negative results.

Colorectal Cancer

18-49 Years	50-65+ Years
Not routine except for patients at high risk. Risk factors include: diagnosis in a first-degree relative; specific genetic syndromes; inflammatory bowel disease; and precancerous polyps. High-risk patients should be screened more frequently using complete colonoscopy at clinician/patient discretion.	Colonoscopy at age 50 and then every 10 years; OR Annual fecal occult blood test (FOBT) plus sigmoidoscopy every 5 years; OR Annual FOBT. Each of the screening strategies has advantages and disadvantages. Screen patients after discussion of the effectiveness, strength of evidence, risks, and complexity of each testing strategy to ensure an informed choice. Discuss benefits and limitations of screening after age 75 in relation to comorbidity based on patient's health status.

Prostate Cancer

18-49 Years	50-69 Years	70+ Years
Screening and routine discussion of screening are not recommended except for patients at high risk for prostate cancer. High-risk men should be provided with the same screening education and screening options as men of age 50-69, but starting at age 40 or above, depending on individual risk.	Screening for prostate cancer with prostate specific antigen (PSA) should not be performed or offered routinely without patient education and informed consent. Providers are encouraged to make men aware that PSA screening is controversial and	Screening and routine discussion of screening are not recommended.

Risk factors include African American ancestry and having a family history of prostate cancer. *Family history of prostate cancer indicates either a brother or father diagnosed with prostate cancer before age 65.*	associated with significant risk of harm, but that screening is an option available to them. Providers are also encouraged to facilitate access information on harms and benefits for men who may be interested in PSA screening. PSA screening may be offered to men who express a clear preference for screening after demonstrating an understanding of the harms and benefits (e.g. through a shared decision making process) and who have a life expectancy of >10 years. For men who express a clear preference for screening after shared decision making: • Screen with PSA every 2 years • For confirmed PSA>4.0 assess/refer for possible prostate biopsy	

The prostate cancer screening guideline was developed by the Massachusetts Prostate Cancer Screening Guideline Panel as part of a contract from the Patient Centered Outcomes Research Institute (PCORI) to the University of Massachusetts Medical School.

Skin Cancer

18-65+ Years
Perform skin exams more frequently at clinician discretion based on risk factors, including: age; personal history of skin cancer or repeated sunburns early in life; family history; certain types and a large number of moles; light skin, light hair, and light eye color; sun-sensitive skin; and chronic exposure to the sun. Educate about skin cancer, including using the ABCDE guidelines to check moles (asymmetry, border, color, diameter, evolving). Counsel to limit exposure to the sun (especially between 10 A.M. and 4 P.M.), to fully cover skin with clothing and hats, and to use sun block (SPF 15 or greater). Discourage use of indoor tanning.

SENSORY SCREENING

Eye Exam

18-39 Years	40-65+ Years
Recommend visit to an eye professional, at least, once, during time period. Recommend screening for glaucoma every 3-5 years in high-risk patients. Risk factors include: African-American ancestry, age, family history of glaucoma, and severe myopia. Screen for glaucoma annually in patients with diabetes.	Recommend screening for glaucoma every 2-4 years. Screen for glaucoma annually in patients with diabetes.

Hearing and Vision Assessment

18-65+ Years
Ask about hearing and vision impairment, and counsel about the availability of treatment when appropriate.

OTHER SCREENINGS

Body Mass Index

18-65+ Years
Screen for obesity at every periodic health evaluation, especially for those with recent weight gain. Consult the CDC's growth and body mass index (BMI) charts. Screen for eating disorders. Ask about body image and dieting patterns. Counsel on the benefits of physical activity and a healthy diet to maintain a desirable weight for height. Offer more-focused evaluation and intensive counseling for adults with BMI> 30kg/m2 to promote sustained weight loss for obese adults.

Cholesterol

18-65+ Years
Screen if not previously tested. Screen every 5 years with lipoprotein profile. If total cholesterol is >200 mg/dl or HDL is <40 mg/dl, a follow-up lipoprotein profile should be performed. More routine screening for patients with high-risk at clinician discretion. High risk includes family history of premature heart disease or hyperlipidemia; hypertension; low HDL; diabetes; tobacco use; age; and weight (BMI>30). If at risk or screened to have high cholesterol and heart disease, counsel on lifestyle changes

including a diet low in saturated fats and high in fiber; weight management; and physical activity.

Diabetes (Type 2)

18-65+ Years
Screen every 3 years, beginning at age 45. Screen more often and beginning at a younger age for those who are overweight and if risk factors are present. Risk factors include: age; first-degree relative with diabetes; physical inactivity; race/ethnicity (African-American, Hispanic, Native American, Asian); high blood pressure (above 140/90mm Hg); history of vascular disease; elevated cholesterol/lipid levels; history of gestational diabetes or birth of a baby > 9 lbs; impaired glucose tolerance; and polycystic ovary syndrome. A fasting blood sugar is the preferred diagnostic test. The 2-hour oral glucose tolerance or HbA1C tests are also acceptable.

Hypertension

18-65+ Years
Screen for high blood pressure at every acute/nonacute medical encounter.

Osteoporosis

18-39 Years	40-64 Years	65+ Years
Counsel about preventive measures, such as dietary calcium and vitamin D intake, weight-bearing exercise, and smoking cessation. Provide bone mineral density (BMD) testing if 10-year fracture risk is equal to or greater than that of a 65 year-old white woman with no additional risk factors.	Counsel about preventive measures, such as dietary calcium and vitamin D intake, weight-bearing exercise, and smoking cessation. Consider risk of osteoporosis in all postmenopausal women. Risk factors include: age; female gender; family/personal history of fractures as an adult; race (Caucasian/Asian); small-bone structure and low body weight (under 127 lbs.); certain menopause or menstrual histories; lifestyle (smoking, little exercise); and certain medications/chronic diseases. Counsel on the risks and benefits of hormonal and non-hormonal therapies. Provide BMD testing for all postmenopausal women who have one or more additional risk	Counsel about preventive measures, such as dietary calcium and vitamin D intake, weight-bearing exercise, and smoking cessation. Provide BMD testing. Counsel elderly patients on specific measures to prevent falls.

	factors for osteoporotic fracture.	

INFECTIOUS DISEASE SCREENING

Sexually Transmitted Infections (Chlamydia, Gonorrhea, Syphilis, and HPV)

18-65+ Years
Advice about risk factors for sexually transmitted infections (STIs) and counsel about effective ways to reduce the risk of infection. For chlamydia and gonorrhea: • Screen all sexually active male and female patients under age 25 annually. Consider urine-based screening for women when a pelvic examination is not performed. • Screen patients age 25 and over annually, if at risk. Risk factors include: inconsistent use of condoms and new or multiple sex partners since last test; history of and/or current sexually transmitted infection; and partner has other sexual partner(s). For syphilis: • Screen if at risk. Risk factors include: history of and/or current infection with another sexually transmitted infection; having more than one sexual partner within the past 6 months; exchanging sex for money or drugs; and men having sex with other men. For HPV: • For age females age 26 and under and males age 21 and under, if not previously vaccinated, counsel patients regarding the schedule for HPV vaccine.

Hepatitis C

18-65+ Years
The American Centre for Disease Control recommends a one-time screening for all adults born between the years 1945-1965, regardless of risk factors. Periodic testing of all patients at high risk. Risk factors include: illicit injection drug use; receipt of blood product for clotting problems before 1990 and/or receipt of a blood transfusion or solid organ transplant before July 1992 (if not previously tested); long-term kidney dialysis; evidence of liver disease; a tattoo or body piercing by nonsterile needle; intravenous drug use; and risky sex practices (not using condoms, multiple sex partners).

HIV

18-65+ Years
The American Centre for Disease Control (CDC|) recommends routine HIV screening for all individuals 18 years of age and older and annual testing for those at increased risk. Counsel about risk factors for HIV infection. Risk factors include: injection-drug users and their sex partners, persons who exchange sex for money or drugs, sex partners of HIV-infected persons, and persons (MSM or heterosexual) who themselves or whose sex partners have had more than one sex partner since their most recent HIV test.

Tuberculosis (TB)

18-65+ Years
Tuberculin skin testing for all patients at high risk. Risk factors include: having spent time with someone with known or suspected TB; having HIV infection; coming from a country where TB is very common; having injected illicit drugs; living in U.S. where TB is more common (e.g., shelters, migrant farm camps, prisons); health care worker; or spending time with others with these risk factors. Determine the need for repeat skin testing by the likelihood of continuing exposure to infectious TB.

GENERAL COUNSELING AND GUIDANCE

Preconception Counseling

18-49 Years	50-65+ Years
Advise all women of child bearing age take to take a daily multivitamin containing .4 mg folate. Encourage scheduling a visit for preconception counseling. Inform patients on the impact of alcohol, drug, tobacco, and environmental exposures in early pregnancy, often before pregnancy is diagnosed. If patient has BMI >30, recommend	N/A

weight loss before becoming pregnant. Counsel pregnant women on the importance of oral health and routine dental care before pregnancy.	

Menopause Management

18-39 Years	40-65+ Year
n/a	Counsel all menopausal women on the management of menopause, including the risks and benefits of hormonal and non-hormonal therapies.

Dementia/Cognitive Impairment

18-49 Years	50-65+ Years
n/a	Observe for possible signs of declining cognitive function in older patients. Evaluate mental status in patients who have problems performing daily activities. Examine patients suspected of having dementia for other causes of changing mental status, including depression, delirium, medication effects, and coexisting medical illnesses.

APPENDIX 1
EATING FOR ENERGY

The concept of energy drinks crept into our diet without letting people know the health implications, just like several individuals on the plus side have resorted to sugar-free drinks in an attempt to watch their weight, without knowing the courtship with medical troubles that may arise.

Most of the energy drinks are truly not energy drinks! You are gradually killing your health and might be too late before you realize it.

"Energy drinks are beverages like Red Bull, Rock Star and Monster, which contain large doses of caffeine and other legal stimulants like guarana and ginseng. The amount of caffeine in an energy drink can range from 75 milligrams to over 200 milligrams per serving. This compares to 34 milligrams in Coke and 55 milligrams in Mountain Dew."
"If a drink advertises no caffeine, the energy comes from guarana, which is the equivalent of caffeine. 5-hour energy drink advertises "no crash," but this claim is referring to no "sugar crash" because the drink has artificial sweeteners." –
Health Education, Brown University.

The 3 big diseases (3BD) Cancer, Diabetes and High Blood Pressure have all been known to be initiated and sustained by certain components found in these drinks.

According to Dr. Joseph Marcola, Aspartame, a sweetener used in the food industry in place of sugar has been found in the production of energy drinks, sugar-free drinks, chewable vitamin C, flavored drinks, etc. and is by far the most dangerous item in the market that is added to foods.

Overwhelming evidence proves it actually promotes weight gain, and is linked to a higher risk of diabetes, headaches, vision problems, high blood pressure, and heart diseases. Aspartame intake is a worse evil when compared with sugar consumption.

According to Dr. Janet Hull, creator of the Aspartame Detox Program, there are over 92 different health side effects associated with aspartame consumption.

Other sweeteners used in energy drinks include Ace-K, sucralose and stevia (stevia is a natural sweetener which is good for other uses outside of energy drinks).

Aside the sweetener, Aspartame, Caffeine is the most common component of energy drinks. Caffeine tolerance varies between individuals. Caffeine has been known to be addictive and is at the root of several medical conditions. Caffeine is also known to cause agitation and restlessness in young people as Cola drinks is also implicated in unstable behavior in kids.

"Dizziness, irritability, increased urination, increased blood pressure, heart palpitations, nausea etc. can all develop at an intolerable dosage on caffeine ." – **The Mayo Clinic**

Consumption of energy drinks poses great danger to pre-existing conditions, especially in cultures where individual's medical history is largely unknown. According to the US National Library of Science, energy drinks cause more forceful heart contractions which could be harmful to people with certain heart conditions.

Individuals with severe and re-current headaches and migraines have also been known to experience relief after stopping the consumption of energy drinks.
Medical News Today recently reported that a compound in energy drinks raises heart risks via gut bacteria.

THOUGHTS & SUGGESTIONS

1. To eat for energy, eat less.

"When you eat too much, your body expends most of its energy on digestion, so, it has less to put towards concentration," - **Rachel Begun, M.S., R.D.**
When your food is rightly prepared, little food gives your body the nourishment it requires.

2. Do you know why there are no depressed monkeys?

Monkeys love bananas. It's a known fact. This is because bananas contain tryptophan, a type of protein that the body converts into serotonin, known to make you relax, improve your mood and generally make you feel happier.

Researchers at Appalachian State University's Human Performance Lab, in the Kannapolis-based North Carolina Research Campus (NCRC), has revealed additional benefits while researching working with cyclists.

"We found that, not only was performance the same whether bananas or sports drinks were consumed, there

were several advantages to consuming bananas. The bananas provided the cyclists with antioxidants not found in sports drinks as well as a greater nutritional boost, including fiber, potassium and Vitamin B6, the study showed. In addition, bananas have a healthier blend of sugars than sports drinks".

When next you think you need energy, go for banana, not energy drink. A note of caution for individuals who are diabetic, as banana can aggravate diabetes.

3. Start the day with this smoothie recipe.

This has been my favorite smoothie recipe since my mentor recommended it. A smoothie is a combo of fruits blended together to form a paste. This particular recipe contains avocado pear, apple and banana. You can use coconut water, coconut milk or carrot juice as your solvent while you blend, using your smoothie maker or your normal kitchen blender.

Avocados are rich in heart-healthy, artery-smoothing unsaturated fats, giving you the best of both worlds - energy, plus less risk of a heart attack and you have also been told that an apple a day, keeps the doctor away.

This gives you a clean and healthy energy than any energy drink can give you. It also offers health benefits for all. Banana is also the sweetener in the combo but individuals with history of diabetes should watch their banana intake.

4. Check out Whole Oats and other Whole grains— The Super Breakfast!

It is an age-long known truth, oats and other whole grains are great for breakfast. They are high in fiber, release fuel for the day's activity and confer several health benefits on the body.

Unfortunately, we have substituted these great meals for "foodless-foods", fast foods and fried foods, like my mentor would say.

According to the American Journal of Clinical Nutrition, in many studies, eating whole grains, such as oats, has been linked to protection against atherosclerosis, ischemic stroke, diabetes, insulin resistance, obesity, and premature death. A new study and accompanying editorial published in the American Journal of Clinical Nutrition explains the likely reasons behind these findings and recommends at least 3 servings of whole grains to be eaten daily.

Wheat bran, for example, which constitutes 15% of most whole-grain wheat kernels, but is virtually non-existent in refined wheat flour, is rich in minerals, antioxidants, lignans, and other phytonutrients—as well as in fiber. There are several health benefits of whole grain which is the reason it is advocated instead of refined/white flour.

You can also drink your oat as milk. Blend your oat using your soyabella machine or your blender, and add a little honey for taste. A glass in the morning is a great starter.

5. What about nut milk?

Any nut can be juiced into milk. This is a great replacement for cow milk and all its attendant issues. Mothers are especially advised to consider this for their family's health.

Nuts like almond, coconut, tigernut (though root crops) give great milk with super healthy benefits. These milks are great starters for your day; they keep you going in the afternoon and get you relaxed after a hard day's work.

You can also get milk from your brown rice (local unpolished rice). Just add a little honey for taste and you may be tempted to forget cow milk for the rest of your life with all the options listed above.

6. Raisins are not just for bread and cakes!

Never knew for a long time the health benefits of raisings, which are dried grape fruits. I sometimes throw them out of their breads and cakes. Raisins are fast energy-giving foods.

Orthodox medicine prescribes the use of glucose-D for people running out of energy for resuscitation, despite the side effects. The use of raisins has been discovered to be more effective than glucose-D.

A 2011 study published in the "Journal of Strength and Conditioning Research" reports that raisins are a feasible energy-boosting alternative to sports jelly beans during high-intensity endurance exercise.

According to Erin Coleman, R.D., L.D. *"Because raisins are rich in carbs, especially natural sugars, they give you a quick boost of energy when you're feeling sluggish -- without weighing you down."*

"Raisins, like all dried fruits, are very good tools for gaining weight in a healthy way, since they are full of fructose and glucose and contain a lot of potential energy. Raisins form an ideal part of a diet for athletes or body builders who need powerful boosts of energy or for those who want to put on weight without accumulating unhealthy amounts of cholesterol." – **Organic Facts.**

Raisings are great to snack on instead of white flour products.

APPENDIX 2
FIBROIDS: DIET & LIFESTYLE OPTIONS

According to the National Uterine Fibroid Foundation (NUFF) of the United States, every 10 minutes, 12 hysterectomies are performed in the US because of uterine fibroids. Possibly as many as 80% of all women have uterine fibroids, while majority usually have no symptoms, 1 in 4 ends up with symptoms severe enough to require treatment.

The more you know about uterine fibroids and your reproductive system, the better you are. As claimed by the NUFF, hysterectomy is certainly a treatment option; it isn't necessarily the only option.

Ten Facts about Fibroids

1. Black women are 2-3 times more likely to present with symptomatic uterine fibroids and will do so at a younger age than the rest of the population of women with uterine fibroids

2. Average age range for fibroids to become symptomatic is between 35 – 50yrs.

3. Asian women have a lower incidence of symptomatic uterine fibroids

4. Obesity is associated with the presence of fibroids (not sure which comes first, fibroid or obesity)

5. Consumption of beef, red meat, dairy products, cow milk, and ham has been associated with uterine fibroids

6. Changes/alteration in a woman's hormone levels may impact fibroid growth

7. Fibroids grow rapidly during pregnancy because of elevated hormonal levels

8. Fibroids shrink after menopause when hormone levels are decreased

9. Estrogen and progesterone play a significant role in fibroid growth

10. Fibroids may increase pregnancy complications and delivery risks.

Symptoms:

- *Heavy Menstrual Bleeding.* The most common symptom is prolonged and heavy bleeding during menstruation. This is caused by fibroid growth bordering the uterine cavity. Menstrual periods may also last longer than normal.

- *Menstrual Pain.* Heavy bleeding and clots can cause severe cramping and pain during menstrual periods.

- *Abdominal Pressure and Pain.* Large fibroids can also cause pressure and pain in the abdomen or lower back that sometimes feels like menstrual cramps.

- *Abdominal and Uterine Enlargement*. As the fibroids grow larger, some women feel them as hard lumps in the lower abdomen. Very large fibroids may give the abdomen the appearance of pregnancy and cause a feeling of heaviness and pressure. In fact, large fibroids are defined by comparing the size of the uterus to the size it would be at specific months during gestation.

- *Pain during Intercourse*. Fibroids can cause pain during sexual intercourse (dyspareunia).

- *Urinary Problems*. Large fibroids may press against the bladder and urinary tract and cause frequent urination or the urge to urinate, particularly when a woman is lying down at night. Fibroids pressing on the ureters (the tubes going from the kidneys to the bladder) may obstruct or block the flow of urine.

- *Constipation*. Fibroid pressure against the rectum can cause constipation.

Fibroid & Reproductive Hormones

The *hypothalamus* (an area in the brain) and the *pituitary gland* regulate the reproductive hormones. The pituitary gland is often referred to as the master gland because of its important role in many vital functions, many of which require hormones.

In women, six key hormones serve as chemical messengers that regulate the reproductive system:

- The hypothalamus first releases the *gonadotropin-releasing hormone (GnRH)* .

- This chemical, in turn, stimulates the pituitary gland to produce *follicle-stimulating hormone (FSH)* and *luteinizing hormone (LH)*.

- *Estrogen, progesterone,* and the male hormone *testosterone* are secreted by the ovaries at the command of FSH and LH and complete the hormonal group necessary for reproductive health.

Estrogen and progesterone appear to play a role in the growth of fibroids.

EFFECT ON PREGNANCY

Fibroids may increase pregnancy complications and delivery risks. These may include:

- Cesarean section delivery

- Breech presentation (baby enters the birth canal upside down with feet or buttocks emerging first)

- Preterm birth

- Placenta previa (placenta covers the cervix)

- Excessive bleeding after giving birth (postpartum hemorrhage)

Anemia:

Anemia, due to iron deficiency, can develop, if fibroids cause excessive bleeding. Oddly enough, smaller fibroids, usually sub-mucous, are more likely to cause abnormally heavy bleeding than larger ones.

Most cases of anemia are mild and can be treated with dietary changes and iron supplements. However, prolonged and severe anemia that is not treated can cause heart problems.

Urinary Tract Infection:

Large fibroids that press against the bladder occasionally result in urinary tract infections. Pressure on the ureters may cause urinary obstruction and kidney damage.

Fibroid and Exposure to Sunlight (Vitamin D Effects):

According to Hormone Matters, fibroids are three to four times more common in African-American women than in white women. Moreover, African-American women are roughly 10 times more likely to be deficient in vitamin D than are white women. Some research suggests that vitamin D can inhibit the growth of human fibroid cells in laboratory cultures.

Recently, researchers from Vanderbilt University Medical Center tested the vitamin D treatment on a strain of rats genetically predisposed to developing fibroid tumors. During the study, rats with uterine fibroids were treated with vitamin D for at least three weeks and similar rats with uterine fibroids were not treated. — Hormone Matters

Thoughts & Suggestions

Meat and Poultry:

Many animals raised for food are given steroids to promote their muscle growth for meat. These steroids leave metabolites available to humans who consume the animal's flesh. According to Skilling and Stringer, although the Food and Drug Administration states that the levels of steroids used to treat animals produced for food is safe, the metabolites, or byproducts of steroids, can be stored in the animals' body fat. Ingesting the metabolites can lead to higher estrogen activity in your body, causing fibroids to grow. If you must eat animal products, choose organically fed and grown without hormones.

Milk, Yogurt and Cheese:

Dairy products, such as milk yogurt and cheese, contain arachidonic acid, which is an essential fatty acid made from linoleic and linolenic acids. When your body receives too much arachidonic acid from animal products, your body releases prostaglandins, which are pro-inflammatory immune system products, according to Skilling and Stringer.

Another point to consider is bovine growth hormone, used to stimulate milk production in post-partum cows. Bovine growth hormone also increases production of a substance called insulin growth factor-1, which stimulates fibroid growth, according to Skilling and Stringer

Canned Foods:

Xenoestrogens are chemical estrogens that are produced when canned food comes in contact with the petroleum-based lining of cans. Xenoestrogens act as weak estrogens in your body and can increase your circulating levels of the estrogen your body makes, according to physician and xenoestrogen expert, Elizabeth Smith, M.D. These xenoestrogens block your body from using estrogen and make it available for your uterine fibroid to grow.

Enriched Processed Foods

Enriched processed foods, such as white bread, regular pasta and white rice, contain very little fiber. Limiting your intake of enriched processed foods in favor of whole-grain breads, whole-grain pastas and brown rice can lessen any constipation and bloating you may experience with uterine fibroids, according to Skilling and Stringer. Enriched processed foods also raise insulin levels faster than foods with fiber. These higher insulin levels increase the availability of estrogen to target uterine-fibroid growth.

Coffee and Tea:

Caffeine isn't directly related to uterine fibroid growth, but it can increase the symptoms you experience. If fatigue is a major issue because of heavy bleeding, drinking coffee and tea will make it worse, because they both decrease the amount of iron your body can absorb. These two drinks contain tannins, which are polyphenols that bind iron, reducing the absorption of the mineral from the foods you eat. Decaffeinated coffees and tea also contain tannins, along with red wine, and all limit iron absorption.

Sugar:

Sugar is the food that most practitioners say to reduce or eliminate if you have fibroids. Sugar is considered a pro-inflammatory food, because it causes your immune system to release antibodies and other hormones that stimulate your body to fight off diseases and foreign materials. Consuming sugar daily over-stimulates your immune system, and these pro-inflammatory responses stay elevated, eventually leading your body to attack itself. Sugar also promotes higher insulin levels, which can lead to lower sex-hormone-binding globulin, which helps your body by binding excess estrogen and deactivating it. The increased estrogen feeds your fibroid tumor and can lead to more severe bleeding, pain, fatigue and other symptoms, according to authors Johanna Skilling and medical doctor Nelson Stringer in "The First Year: Fibroids."

Printed in Great Britain
by Amazon